Carpal Tunnel Symptoms and Treatments

Dan Spada

Carpal Tunnel Symptoms and Treatments
by Dan Spada

ISBN 978-1-926917-23-8

Printed in the United States of America

TABLE OF CONTENTS

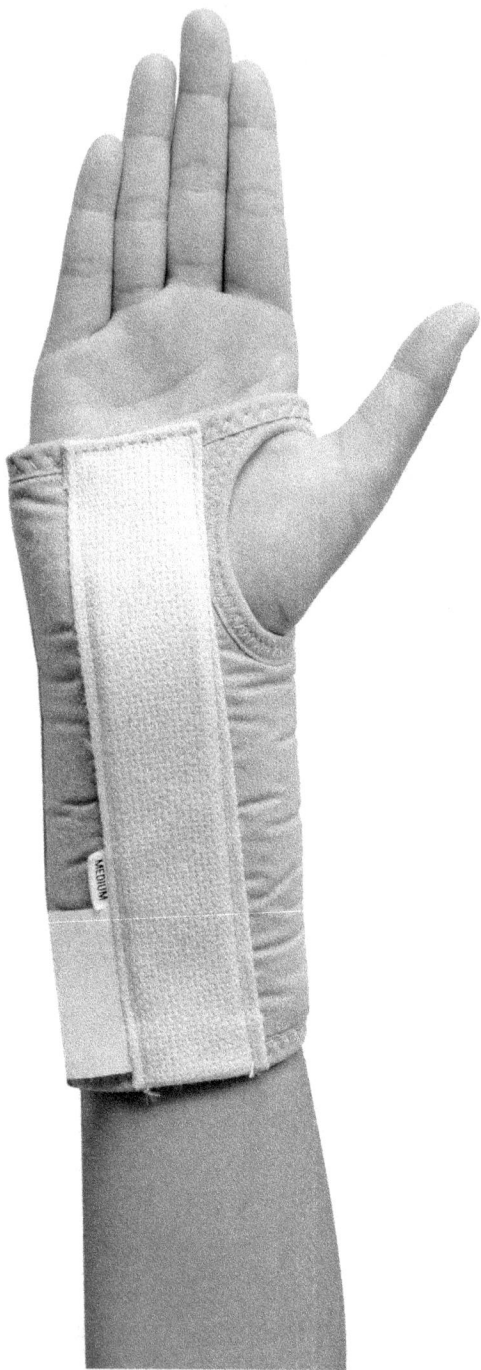

Introduction

Around the world many people suffer from a condition known as carpal tunnel syndrome or CTS. This condition involves the nerves which control the function of both the hand and the fingers. Resulting in tingling, numbness and pain, this is a very serious condition that can leave an individual in severe discomfort and can even affect life activities, including the ability to work.

Understanding carpal tunnel syndrome and the treatments that are available for this condition is absolutely essential in order for an individual to recover and be able to enjoy previous activities and hobbies as well as an improved quality of life.

Today, there are actually many treatments and options that are available for curing this condition, but it is essential for an individual who suffers from this painful condition to be well educated and informed about both the condition as well as the options that are available for treatment.

In this guide, you will not only learn about the condition itself, but you will also learn about what is involved in the treatment options that are available so that you will be prepared to make the most well informed decision possible regarding which treatment option is best for you and your situation as well as your lifestyle.

Are you ready to get rid of carpal tunnel syndrome?

Let's get started!

Understanding Carpal Tunnel Syndrome

Before we can begin to examine the treatment options that are available for carpal tunnel syndrome, it is important to first examinee the nature and background of this condition.

What Exactly is Carpal Tunnel Syndrome or CTS?

Carpal tunnel syndrome, often referred to as CTS, is a condition that involves the major nerves of the hand and fingers. These nerves control the function of the fingers and hands and together are referred to as the median nerve. When these nerves become compressed inside a tunnel within the wrist, the result is the symptoms that are most commonly associated with carpal tunnel syndrome. These symptoms can include:

- Tingling
- Numbness
- Pain
- A 'funny' feeling in the hand, wrist or fingers

The carpal tunnel is a small passageway that is located inside the wrist. Several small bones inside the wrist form the sides as well as the bottom of this tunnel. The roof of the tunnel is formed by a ligament that is known as the transverse carpal ligament. This ligament arches over the small bones. The median nerve is located inside the tunnel and is responsible for conducting impulses sent by the brain all the way down to the fingers and the arm. The tendons for the finger flexor muscles are also located inside the tunnel. These tendons are responsible for making it possible for the fingers to bend. There are also veins and arteries inside the tunnel as well.

The majority of the feeling in the hand is supplied by the median nerve. This is especially true for the index and middle fingers as well as the thumb. The feeling for the outer side of the hand as well as the thumb part of the palm is supplied by the median nerve as well. The median nerve also controls movement of the tendons that work to bend the fingers, making it possible for you to grasp objects with your hand as well as pinch.

CTS Symptoms

The symptoms of CTS tend to appear gradually. These symptoms may include the following:

- Tingling, numbness or a burning sensation in the fingers and thumb. The index and middle fingers may be especially affected.
- Pain in the wrists and hands
- Loss of gripping strength or dexterity
- Difficulty in performing routine tasks such as holding a cup, washing one's hands, vacuuming, holding a telephone, driving, etc.
- Pain in the shoulder and arm
- Swelling of the hand. May increase at nighttime.

One of the surest signs of carpal tunnel syndrome

is when the symptoms become so severe that the individual is awakened at night from sleep due to pain or tingling in the hand. Symptoms often tend to worsen at night due to the way the hand is commonly positioned while sleeping. Some individuals have found relief by holding their hand either high or low and shaking their hand. Rubbing the hands together or soaking the hand in warm water may also help when such symptoms appear.

The Cause of CTS

At this time, the exact cause of carpal tunnel syndrome remains unknown. In most cases, there is no obvious cause. It is known that any condition or situation which restricts the amount of space present in the carpal tunnel can cause the median nerve to become compressed. Such situations and conditions may include:

- Injuries, including prior wrist fractures
- Medications that have caused fluid retention. This includes oral contraceptives or birth control pills.
- Hormonal changes as well as conditions that result in fluid retention, such as pregnancy. When CTS occurs during pregnancy, it typically resolves itself within six weeks of delivery
- Medical disorders that result in constricted blood vessels, like Raynaud's disease
- Medical conditions that result in fluid

retention or inflammation, including diabetes, rheumatoid arthritis, Lyme disease and hypothyroidism

Additionally, it should be understood that both smoking as well as obesity can result in the development of carpal tunnel syndrome because this causes a constriction of the blood vessels as well as increased pressure on the nerves within the wrist.

Carpal Tunnel Syndrome and Repetitive Strain Injury

During the 1970s many conditions which involved the upper tends and joints were attributed to repetitive strain injury or RSI. It was thought that such injuries resulted from prolonged overuse of the upper extremities as a result of repetitive motions of the hand, elbows and fingers that were too fast.

It is believed by some researchers that overuse of the wrist might result in carpal tunnel syndrome. Not all physicians accept this idea. Repetitive strain injury has gradually become less recognized as a cause of the symptoms of carpal tunnel syndrome.

It is primarily assumed by those doctors who still associate the symptoms of carpal tunnel syndrome with RSI that an unnatural bending or prolonged overuse can inflame the protective layer of the tendons. This sheath is known as the synovial sheath and can result in swelling. When the tendons are swollen, pressure may be placed on the median nerve in the carpal tunnel. As a result, the nerve impulses may be disrupted and the normal functioning of the nerve may be impaired as a result.

Repetitive strain injuries have become the most rapid growing category of occupational related injuries. They are also leading cause of occupational related illness, accounting for more than 64% of all workplace illnesses, an increase of some 33%.

Activities that Can Result in CTS

In some instances, certain activities can trigger CTS. This includes poor posture, such as slouching and working in a position that causes the wrists to bend upward, outward or inward. Such activities may include:

- Cutting
- Using vibrating tools
- Knitting, sewing or crocheting
- Using hand tools for twisting or turning (wrenches, screwdrivers)
- House cleaning
- Bicycling
- Playing a stringed instrument
- Typing
- Pointing and clicking using a computer mouse

Who is Most at Risk for CTS?

The U.S. Bureau of Labor Statistics reported cases of CTS most frequently in the following occupations and industries:

- Knit underwear mills
- Meat packing plants
- Motor vehicles
- Poultry slaughtering and processing
- Household laundry equipment manufacturing

Interestingly, homemakers are actually more commonly treated for CTS than individuals in the above industries.

Conditions that Can Result in Similar Symptoms

In some instances the symptoms associated with carpal tunnel syndrome can also be mimicked by other medical conditions and disorders, including:

- Circulation disorders
- Arthritis of the hand, wrist or neck
- Previous injuries to the wrist
- Nerve disorders
- Tendonitis of the wrist

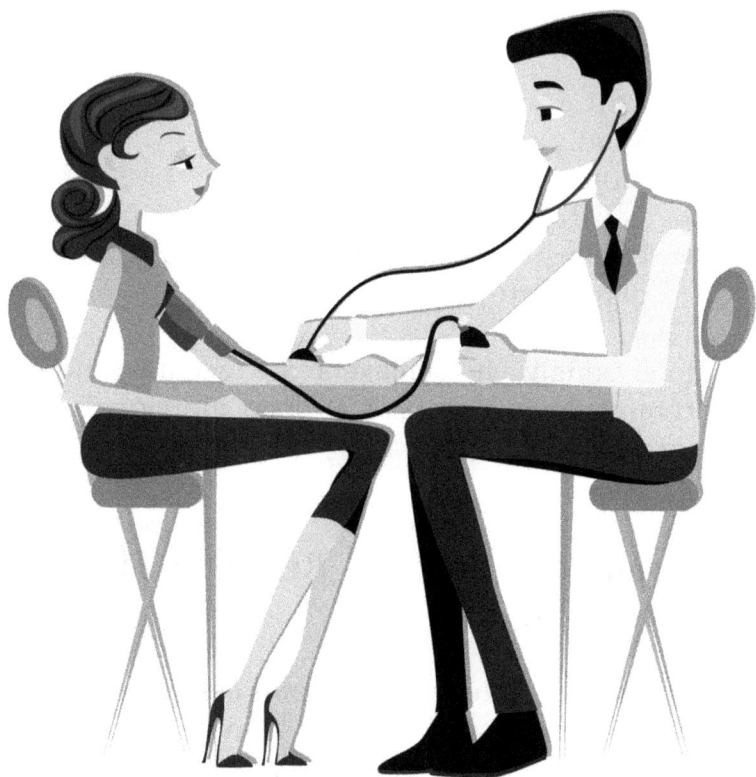

Diagnosing CTS

In order to diagnose carpal tunnel syndrome, a physician will take a medical history, including information about the following:

- Symptoms experienced and activities that seem to trigger symptoms
- Duration of symptoms
- What seems to improve or worsen symptoms
- Overall medical background

In addition, the physician will also examine your wrists, elbows, hands, neck and shoulder in order to check for problems such as nerve compression. He or she may also perform a physical exam to check for other medical problems as well. For example, the physician may tap your wrist directly over the median nerve in order to determine whether this reproduces the associated symptoms. This is known as a Tinel test.

He or she may also gently hold the wrist in a forward bent position for 30 to 60 seconds in order to determine whether this triggers symptoms. This is known as the Phalen test.

The physician may also use light stroking motions or pinpricks using a pin to determine whether any portion of the have reduced or lost sensitivity. This can be a sign of nerve damage.

If you think that you may have carpal tunnel syndrome, you may wish to consult your family doctor or consult an orthopedist or neurologist. A physician that specializes in occupational medicine is also a good choice. If it is determined that surgery is required, an orthopedic surgeon or hand surgeon will be necessary.

Specialized Tests

In some instances it may not be clear whether the symptoms that a patient experiences are associated with the median nerve or perhaps somewhere higher in the arm. The symptoms could potentially be linked to a problem with the nerves within the hand or even the nerves in the neck, resulting in tingling and pain that radiates down into the hand.

Specialized tests can help to resolve any uncertainty. Such tests include:

Nerve Conduction Test

This is a test that is used to determine whether the transmission in the nerve has been reduced as a result of nerve damage. A physician will place electrodes on the wrist and hand. Small electric shocks will then be applied to the nerves within the wrist, forearm and fingers in order to determine whether the nerve messages are being properly conducted.

Electromyography

In severe cases, the muscles that are supplied by the nerve may demonstrate abnormal electrical activity. A doctor will insert a very fine wire into the muscle within the affected area for a brief period of time. Electrical activity can then be displayed on a monitor for the doctor to evaluate.

X-Rays

X-rays of the neck and wrist may also be taken in order to rule out any previous fractures or arthritis. It should be noted that x-rays alone cannot be used to diagnose CTS.

Magnetic Resonance Imaging (MRI)

This test can be used to determine if there are any structural abnormalities of the wrist that could contribute to carpal tunnel syndrome.

Non-Surgical Treatments for CTS

Naturally, one of the most common questions about CTS is how it can be effectively treated. It should be understood that if there is continued compression of the nerve this can result in symptoms that become increasingly severe. Ultimately, nerve damage can be caused and some of the functions of the hand can be permanently impaired. Therefore, it is important to seek treatment rather than to just let it go and assume that the condition will improve on its own without intervention.

Proper treatment of CTS can help to manage and cure CTS as well as prevent permanent disability from occurring. The types of conventional treatment that are available may depend upon the severity of the condition. The following measures may be used, based on the severity of symptoms:

- Resting the wrist for a time period through the use of a wrist splint
- Physical therapy
- Modifying work habits and activities
- Modifying your work station through the use of ergonomics
- Using anti-inflammatory medications
- Using diuretics
- Steroid injections in the wrist
- Treating a related condition that may result in CTS symptoms
- Alternative treatments

Your physician may also recommend the use

of specific exercises in order to stretch as well as lengthen the wrist. As a last resort, if other treatments are not effective, surgery may also be considered.

Wrist Splints

A wrist splint is a device that is used to prevent the wrist from bending. The use of a wrist splint is meant to prevent pressure from being applied to the median nerve. The palm is prevented from bending forward. There are actually several different types of splints that can be used:

- Neutral splints-meant to keep the wrist perfectly straight
- Cock-up splints-holds the wrist in a position that is slightly extended and bent somewhat upwards. These splints can be particularly useful at night as well as well driving and during other activities in which the wrist would otherwise be bent forward.
- Occupational specific splints-These splints can be custom made for individuals involved in certain jobs

It should be noted that a splint should not be worn all day as this can result in further weakness of the muscle as well as worsening of the symptoms. The splint should be removed for a period of time every four to six hours.

Many people find they can relieve symptoms

by just wearing the splint at night, although you should recognize that your symptoms and the condition will improve at a far faster rate if you wear the splint more often. There should be no concerns about growing dependent upon it.

Keep in mind that it will likely take you a few nights to become accustomed to wearing it. Eventually you will get used to wearing it and it won't bother you as much, but in the beginning you may have to work your way up to wearing it for longer periods of time.

Wearing the splint to bed will assist in keeping your wrist in a neutral position and make it possible for the structures in the wrist to rest properly. Think of it this way; when you bend a garden hose, the water flow is cut off. When the hose is straightened out, the water flow resumes. The same is also true for your wrist and the nerves present inside your wrist.

During sleep, it is only natural to bend the wrists in a fetal position. This results in kinking up the nerves. If you are able to straighten out the wrist, you can achieve proper nerve conduction. Over time, you will likely find that your symptoms improve.

Some people do decide to continue wearing the splint at night indefinitely. There is certainly nothing wrong with that. Other individuals elect to gradually wean themselves off wearing the splint. This is an entirely personal decision and is one which should be based on your own experiences.

It is also imperative that the splint fit properly so that all of the fingers are able to move freely. In most instances, the physician that diagnoses you with CTS can provide a splint, but if that is not the case you can pick one up at a discount store or pharmacy. They are usually located in the health and beauty section. Common brands of splints include Futuro and Ace. They are commonly called wrist splints or carpal tunnel splints. These splints feature a metal on the bottom and can be wrapped all the way around the wrist.

Before purchasing the splint, it is a good idea to try it on while you are still at the store or pharmacy. This is important because you need to be certain that the splint fits well. If it is not comfortable, you will be less likely to wear it and therefore will not receive any benefit from it. Most splints cost between $10 and $15.

Better quality splints can usually be obtained at an orthopedic store. You can usually find such stores near hospital. These splints are going to be more expensive and can cost up to $35. They do tend to fit better; however, and you can receive assistance from a trained professional in selecting the proper splint. In some instances, your health insurance company may even cover the cost, although you will probably need a prescription from your doctor.

You might also consider purchasing a wrist splint online. There are certainly plenty of options available for doing so online, but you should consider the fact that this does not give you the opportunity to try on the splint before buying it to make sure it fits well.

Physical Therapy

In some instances, physical therapy may also be appropriate to treat CTS. A physical therapist can work with you to custom design an exercise regimen to help relieve the symptoms. Physical therapy can also involves measures that are meant to relieve pain. Such pain relief measures may include:

- Ice packs
- Moist heat
- Ultrasound through the use of placing electrodes on the skin to block pain

Anti-Inflammatory Medications

Anti-inflammatory medications, which are also known as non-steroidal anti-inflammatory drugs or NSAIDs are also commonly used to manage the symptoms of CTS. Many such medications can be purchased over the counter. Such medications include naproxen and ibuprofen. COX-2 is a relatively new anti-inflammatory drug that was introduced just a few years ago and is reported to have fewer side effects than other medications, but has since been withdrawn from the market because it was determined that it could result in serious cardiovascular side effects that had been previously unrecognized. Celebrex is still available.

It should be noted that the use of NSAIDs can result in stomach upset. Prolonged use of such medications can also cause stomach bleeding. Taking food with these medications can help to minimize such side effects.

Diuretics

Diuretics are also commonly known as water pills and work to reduce fluid retention within the body. They may help symptoms of CTS in some cases due to the fact that excess fluid can aggravate symptoms. For example, in women, symptoms may become more severe during their menstrual cycle.

Steroid Injections

Steroid injections may also sometimes be used in the wrist if simpler measures have not produced results. It should be noted that such injections are not thought to cause the same undesirable side effects that are associated with the long term use of steroids. Relief provided by such injections can be permanent or temporary.

When CTS is caused by the presence of rheumatoid arthritis, oral steroids may be of some help, but they should not be taken when CTS is caused by excess fluid or repetitive strain injury. Oral steroids must be carefully monitored.

Alternative Treatments

Alternative treatments can be helpful in some cases when used in combination with conventional treatments.

Cold Laser Therapy

This treatment is non-invasive and utilizes a low energy or 'cold' laser light to penetrate the skin as well as the soft tissue. The process is meant to simulate the nerve and increase circulation within the wrist.

Acupuncture

This is an ancient Chinese treatment that has been used for hundreds of years to treat various conditions. A trained acupuncturist inserts very fine needles into various points on the body. It is thought that energy flows throughout the body along paths known as meridians. If the energy is interrupted, the result can be illness or pain. Needles are inserted in order to stimulate the flow of energy. There may be some discomfort as the needles are inserted, but most people do find some relief when the process is properly performed.

Vitamin B6

This vitamin is also known as pyridoxine and it is thought by some researchers that the use of it can relieve CTS. It should be noted that it is not advised to exceed 200 milligrams per day. More than this amount can result in nerve damage. Also, keep in mind that any vitamin supplementation should be an important part of a balanced diet.

Magnetic Therapy

It is thought by some people that magnets that have between a 550 and 850 gauss can stimulate the flow of blood as well as provide pain relief. Gauss is a unit of measurement for the strength of a magnet. The side of the magnet possesses a negative polarity that is used to fasten against the skin using tape or with a wrap or splint.

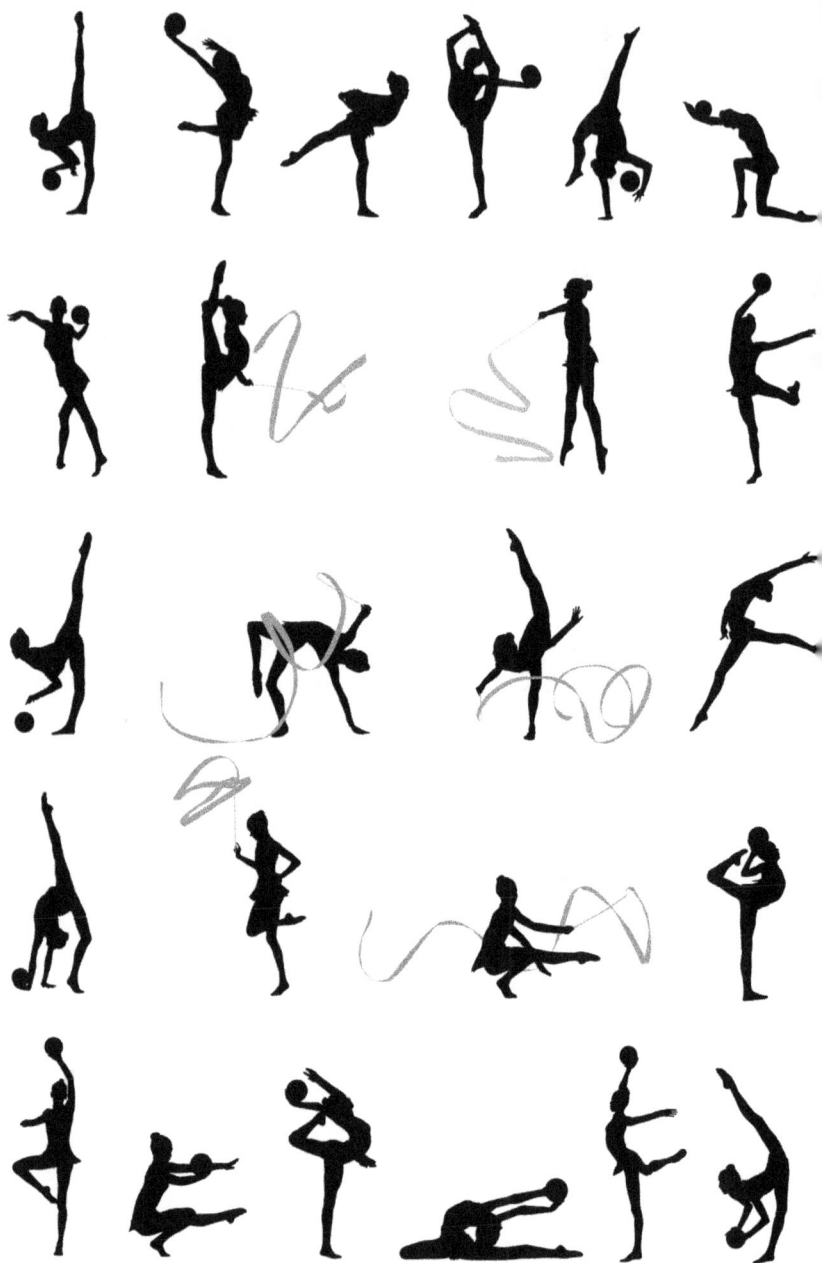

Exercises and Therapeutic Measures for Preventing and Managing CTS

There are many things that you can do to relieve some of the symptoms that are commonly associated with CTS. One of the most important things that you can do is reduce the swelling. This is crucial before you attempt any type of exercise because it is usually the swelling that is present within the carpal tunnel that presents some of the most common problems.

Contrast Baths

This is perhaps one of the most effective techniques you can use at home in order to reduce swelling. In order to use this technique, you will need either two bowls or two sinks in which to place water. One will need to be hot enough to produce steam and the other will need to be cold and filled with two trays of ice. You should also have a timer nearby so that you can time the amount of time you have your hand in the water.

You will start off in the hot water and have your hand in the water for four minutes. Immediately switch to the cold water and keep it there for one minute. Now, switch back to the hot water for four minutes then back to the cold water for one minute. Repeat this twice and make sure that you end with four minutes in the hot water.

Keep in mind that you may need to add more ice or heat to the bowls of water in order to maintain the correct temperatures. Be prepared for the fact that the hot water may feel just fine but the cold water is likely to sting.

This technique is meant to force the blood vessels in the hand and wrist to dilate, which will force out the swelling. It is not unusual to notice that pain is immediately relieved following a contrast bath.

Exercises

Exercises can be used to prevent as well as to manage the symptoms associated with CTS. Keep in mind that it is important for a physical therapist to always approve in exercise or physical therapy plan before you start.

You should also know that such exercises are not intended to be used as a substitute for the examination and consultation by a qualified specialist. If you have an acute injury, you should not attempt such exercise.

Also, remember that you should always ice the affected area immediately before beginning any exercise.

There are many different exercises that can be used to prevent and treat CTS symptoms.

Wrist Range of Motion

This exercise can be performed by placing the

forearm on a table so that the wrist is off the edge of the table and the palm is facing downward. Bend the hand downward as far as possible and then bend it upward. Repeat five to ten times.

Wrist Range of Motion #2

Place the forearm and the entire hand on a table with the palm flat on the top of the table. Turn the wrist so that the back of the hand is flat against the tabletop. Repeat five to ten times.

Flexed Forearm Stretch

Extend the affected arm straight out in front of your body without raising the shoulders. Bend the wrist downward using your free hand, slowly and gently. Make sure that the fingers are kept over the knuckles of the hand that is best instead of over the fingers. You should be able to feel the forearm muscles stretch. Hold this position for ten seconds. Repeat five to ten times.

Flexed Forearm Stretch #2

Repeat the above exercise, except this time make a fist first and then bend the wrist downward. Hold for ten seconds. Repeat five to ten times.

Forearm Stretch #3

Stretch the forearm muscles so that the arms are extended out to the side and straight. The palms should be facing backward. Bend the wrists back.

Hold for ten seconds. Repeat five to ten times.

Forearm Stretch #4

Extend the arm straight outward in front of you with the palm facing outward. Use your free hand on the underside of the knuckles and then press it backward toward the body. Make sure you do not raise your shoulders. You should be able to feel a slight stretch in the underside of the forearm. Hold for ten seconds. Repeat five to ten times.

Tendon Glide

Begin with a relaxed hand. The fingers should be straight. Make a fist. Now, slide the fingertips to the base of the hand, making sure the thumb is straight. Next, glide the fingers upward so that a hook is formed. Repeat five to ten times.

Neck Stretch

Begin by sitting or standing with the head facing forward. Tilt your head downward to the right as much as you can and then hold for five seconds. Place the right hand between the neck and shoulder joint. This is known as the left trapezius muscle and can help to increase the stretch. Reverse for the other side. Repeat three to five times.

Shoulder Shrug Rotation

Begin by standing with your arms at your sides.

Shrug your shoulders upwards toward your ears. Now, squeeze your shoulders backward, stretching them down and then rolling them forward. Make sure that you do this slowly. Repeat three to five times.

Pectoral Stretch

Begin by standing in either a corner or doorway. Rest the forearms on the doorframe, with your arms bent at a 90 degree angle. Lean forward until you feel a stretch inside the chest muscles. Make sure that you do not arch your back. Hold this position for 20 seconds and then repeat five times.

Full Fist Exercise

Begin by having your fingers completely straight. Take your hand and bring it into a position with a full fist. The fingertips should be curled all of the way under. Return your hand to the original straight position. Repeat ten to fifteen times.

Straight Fist Exercise

Begin with the fingers straight. Bring the fingertips down so that they touch the palm of the hand. The fingertips should not be curled under. Instead, the pads of the fingertips should brush the palm. Return to the original straight position. Repeat ten to fifteen times.

The Bugle

Begin with all of the fingers straight. Pretend you are playing the bugle, using each finger separately. Perform the same motion with each finger at least ten times before you move on to the next finger.

Do not be surprised if you notice some pain or a strange feeling when performing these exercises. If you reach a position which is painful or uncomfortable, start back at the first position and then repeat it. Remember that it is never helpful to push beyond the point of comfort.

Decompression Movements

These exercises or movements are meant to stretch the carpal tunnel so that the nerves will have plenty of room to breathe and will no longer be compressed. These movements should be performed at least three times per day.

- Begin with the arms held out straight in front of you. The wrists should be straight. Make a tight fist using both hands. Hold this position for five seconds.

- Bend the wrists, with the hands still fisted. Bend as far as you can and then hold for five seconds.

- Release the fisted position and allow your wrists to straighten out. Hold for five seconds.

- Now, hang both arms down to the sides and shake them.

- Repeat this series of movements ten times and perform a minimum of three times per day.

Resting your Hands and Wrists

It is also important to make sure that you give your hands plenty of time to rest. It is important during this phase to make sure that you back off from whatever activity it is that has been aggravating or irritating your symptoms. This should be done for a few weeks.

During this time you need to cease excessive typing, gripping, gardening, etc. Whatever it is that has triggered your symptoms, you need to back away from. You should also make sure you are not using scissors or tools that vibrate excessively.

The goal of this is to give your tendons ample time to heal. It is quite difficult for that to occur if you are still continuing to perform the same motions that have aggravated your symptoms in the first place. Give your hands ample time to rest and heal. Overuse is what commonly causes tendons to become irritated as well as swollen.

Modifying Work Habits

Modifying your work habits can be an excellent way to help relieve some of the symptoms associated with CTS. Make sure that you take frequent breaks. When possible take a break every thirty minutes, but at least take a break every hour and a half. During your break, make a point to get up from your work area, walk around and stretch.

- When possible, try to rotate tasks so that you are not continually performing the same tasks over and over.

- Make sure that you maintain the proper posture. Ergonomics can assist you with this.

- When you hold an object, be sure that you utilize your entire hand and not just the thumb or fingers.

- Select tools that are well-balanced and are easy to hold. Along the same lines, make sure that any cutting instruments, such as scissors and knives, are sharp.

- If you use compressed air tools, be sure to check them from time to time. Too much pressure can cause injury to the wrists and hands.

Keep mind when performing any exercise or therapeutic program to relieve the symptoms of CTS that the longer you have had symptoms, the longer it will take for you to recover.

This does not mean that it is impossible, but you should be prepared for the fact that you very well ma need to try these techniques for at least a month before you will be able to reasonably determine whether they are working.

You should also be aware of the fact that these techniques may not relieve your symptoms 100%. You may notice after performing these exercises and techniques that you are not as disturbed by the pain at night or that your hands are not as painful as they once were, but that you do continue to experience some symptoms from time to time.

Is it Working?

We have already discussed this, but it is important to note in greater detail that you should not expect immediate results from these techniques. You must be prepared for the fact that recovering from CTS can be a slow process. It is one hat does require patience as well as continued and consistent effort.

There are some people who may notice a lessening of their symptoms within just a few days of beginning this type of program, but for the most part, you will not notice any change until at least two to three weeks. Even after three or so weeks, the changes may not be significant, so you should be prepared for this.

At a minimum, you should be prepared to give this type of program at least eight weeks in order to determine whether it is working and is effective for you before you stop. A full eight weeks of performing the techniques and exercises described here should be enough time for you to notice at least some degree of improvement in the symptoms you previously experienced.

If you do not notice any improvement at all, you should see your doctor to determine whether other treatment methods may be appropriate for your situation. Such treatment options may include surgery or formal therapy.

Formal therapy can involve other techniques that cannot be as easily performed at home. This is because in some cases a special machine or equipment may be needed. If you need to locate a therapist, you can look online at www.asht.org.

In order to determine whether surgery is appropriate for your particular situation, your physician may also wish to perform tests to determine the severity of your condition.

The following worksheet can also assist you in determining whether surgery may be appropriate for your particular situation. Be sure to discuss it with your physician.

Carpal Tunnel Surgery Worksheet

Once you complete the following worksheet, you should have an idea of how you feel about the possibility of carpal tunnel syndrome.

Circle the answer that best applies to you.

I have consistently followed the instructions prescribed by physician for at least 3 months.	Yes	No	Unsure
Non-surgical treatment is improving my symptoms.	Yes	No	Unsure
I have severe pain, numbness, or weakness that makes daily activities difficult	Yes	No	Unsure
I am disabled by carpal tunnel syndrome.	Yes	No	NA*
I must severely limit my daily activities because of my condition.	Yes	No	NA
I am concerned I will develop median nerve damage	Yes	No	Unsure
I have been diagnosed with median nerve damage.	Yes	No	Unsure
I feel comfortable with the idea of having surgery.	Yes	No	Unsure
I have carpal tunnel syndrome that has caused weakness, pain and numbness for more than a year.	Yes	No	Unsure

Use the following space to list any other concerns you have about this decision that may be important.

Surgical Treatment for CTS

If you have tried to heal through exercises and therapy and you have still not seen any improvement during the last couple of months, then you may need to consider surgery. For most people, surgery is considered only as a last resort and you should always make sure that you thoroughly discuss this option with a physician.

Finding a Doctor

One of the key steps will be to select a doctor. Many people never realize that there are actually several options that are available when it comes to choosing one to perform your carpal tunnel syndrome. Options include:

- Neurosurgeon
- Orthopedic surgeon
- Plastic surgeon

It is always a good idea to ask for references and get the opinions of people you may know who have had this procedure performed. Regardless of which type of specialist you choose, make sure you schedule plenty of time to have a consultation with the doctor so that you can discuss the procedure and the impact it may have on your daily activities and work.

You should be aware that surgery can help to abolish the symptoms associated with CTS. There are some instances; however, in which this may not be the case. This could happen if the nerve has experienced damage that is irreversible over a long period of time. If there is a loss of sensation and the nerve is no longer able to function in a normal manner, then the symptoms will likely persist.

You should also be aware of the fact that the tingling and pain that are associated with CTS will usually disappear not long after the surgery. Numbness within the fingers and the palm could take longer to vanish.

Types of Surgery

There are two primary types of carpal tunnel syndrome surgery. They are:

- Open carpal tunnel release surgery
- Endoscopic or keyhole surgery

The type of surgery that you opt for may depend upon your particular situation and the procedure that your doctor feels is best and will provide you with the optimal chance for full recovery.

Open Carpal Tunnel Release Surgery

The idea behind this procedure is to increase the amount of space in the carpal tunnel so that there is no longer any pressure on the median nerve. It is a fairly simple procedure and can usually be performed on an outpatient basis.

This procedure can be performed using a local anesthetic, regional anesthetic or general anesthetic.

- A local anesthetic involves an injection of a substance that will numb the hand where the incision will be made.

- A regional anesthetic utilizes a numbing substance that is injected into the upper arm in order to numb the whole arm.

- A general anesthesia place the patient completely under so they are asleep during the procedure.

This type of procedure involves dividing the ligament that forms the roof of the carpal tunnel. This will make it possible for the nerve to pass through the tunnel freely without any compression. An incision approximately 1 ½ to 2 inches in length will be made in the palm and extend up toward the wrist.

The ligament will then be exposed and divided carefully. This will allow the median nerve to be visible in the tunnel. The nerve will be inspected to make sure that it is free and there are no obstructions. The incision will then be closed.

After Surgery

Following the procedure, a dressing of bandages and a splint may be used. A plaster cast may also be used in some cases for up to two weeks. It is important for the hand to be elevated in order to reduce swelling. A sling can be worn for additional comfort. You should avoid leaning on our hand or having your hand hang down as this will increase swelling.

It is a good idea to remove your arm from the sling every few hours so that you can move your shoulder and elbow to prevent them from becoming stiff. Make sure that you move your fingers regularly as well.

You will need to take care that you do not get the dressing wet. If you need to bathe, cover the dressing using a plastic bag. Sutures can usually be removed within a week to ten days. In some instances, absorbable sutures may be used, which eliminates the need to have them removed.

After the sutures have been removed, the surgeon will usually tell you that you need to move your hand and fingers. You can then begin exercises based on gripping at this point. A supervised hand therapy program may also be prescribed. Massaging the scar with cream or oil may also be helpful.

Recovery

You may be able to return to work within two to eight weeks. The timeframe will depend upon the severity of your condition, the type of surgery that was performed, your progress in rehab and the nature of your work. If you perform work that involves repetitive motions your recovery may take longer and could last up to ten weeks.

Endoscopic or Keyhole Surgery

This is a relatively new procedure that involves using a small incision at the wrist which makes it possible for the surgeon to place a fiber-optic tool in an endoscope and in the carpal tunnel. Small instruments are then used to divide the ligament. The surgeon will view the carpal tunnel are as well as the median nerve on a video monitor.

There are numerous advantages to endoscopic surgery. These benefits include the fact that recovery time is usually much faster. In addition, the scar is also smaller. Not all surgeons are experienced with using this procedure due to the fact that it is a newer type of surgery.

Recovery

You should know that the recovery period following this procedure can depend upon the exact type of procedure that is performed as well as the severity of the damage and your own medical history and health. You should also recognize that your recovery period can also depend upon exactly what it is that you need to do in order to return to normal activity.

As a general rule of thumb, you should anticipate a minimum of several weeks of stiffness and soreness. The scar tissue will usually begin to build up around the area where the incision was made. You may also notice that it may be hard to lean onto your hand without feeling some discomfort.

After the surgery has been completed, you should ask your surgeon to provide you with a referral for therapy in order to make sure that you get on the right track for proper healing.

Bilateral Carpal Tunnel Release Surgery

If you are experiencing symptoms in both hands, your physician may recommend having a procedure performed on both hands. This is known as a bilateral carpal tunnel release.

If that is the case, you may seriously want to consider spacing the surgeries out a month from one another at a minimum. This will provide your body with plenty of time to rest from the first procedure before attempting a second procedure.

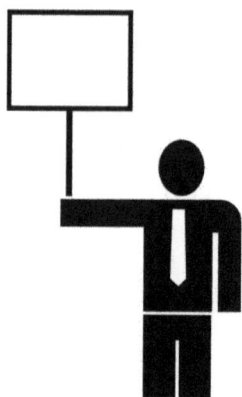

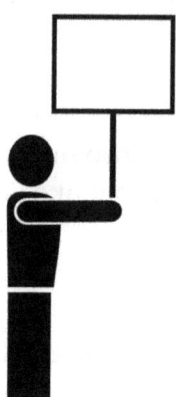

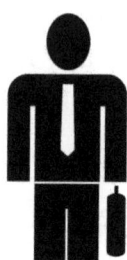

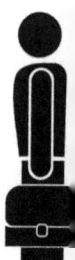

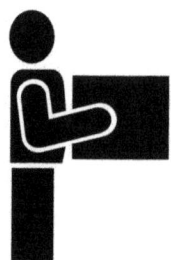

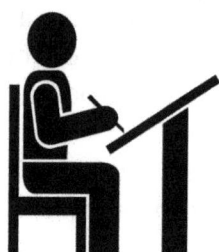

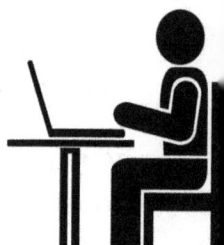

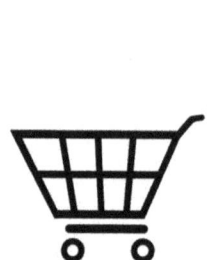

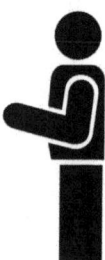

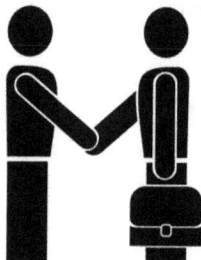

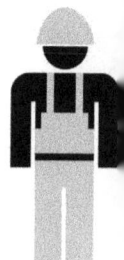

Occupational Considerations

Many people never realize that the symptoms they have experienced could be related to something they are doing at their job. In the event that you have a data entry job, office job or some other type of job that is computer based, it is possible that the problems you are experiencing are related to repetitive stress. If you think that is the case, you should see your doctor and have him perform an exam to determine whether the condition is related to RSI or CST.

In the event that it is determined that your injuries are work related it is possible that you may be able to qualify for a workman's compensation claim. If it is determined that your injuries are not work related you can always consider using a therapy program and then considering using surgery later on if the therapy does not relieve your symptoms.

Remember as well that it is always important for you to evaluate the layout of your work area to determine whether there are any changes that can be made to make it more comfortable for you. For example, look at your computer to see whether it is at eye level. What about the items you use most often? Are they near you on your desk?

Do you frequently have to strain your neck in order to hold the phone to your ear? How are your feet positioned? Are they directly on the floor in front of you?

Re-arranging your workspace may help you to receive some relief from the symptoms you have been experiencing.

Remember that it is important to get up and walk around once every hour so that you can stretch your arms and neck. Also stretch your shoulder blades together so that you will have the correct posture when you are working. Correct posture is essential to full recovery.

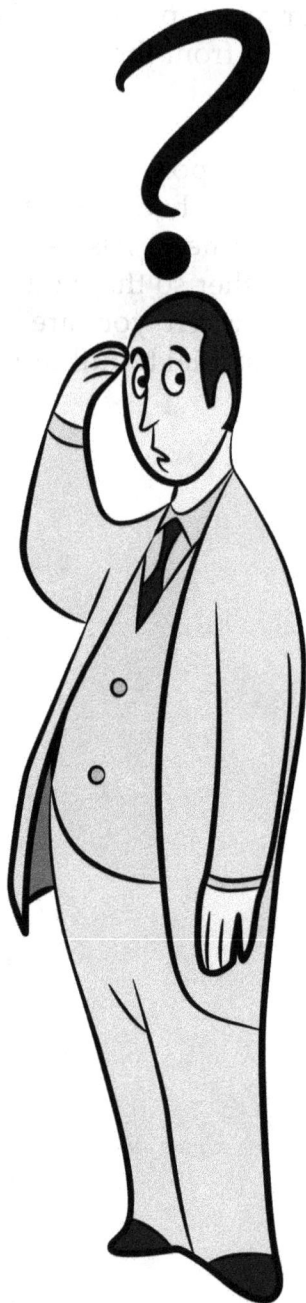

What to do if it is not CTS

If you have found that the symptoms you are experiencing are not those that have been described as associated with CTS then it is possible that you are experiencing a completely different condition. There are other possible symptoms that could be related to different conditions, such as:

- A burning sensation in the thumb
- Finger or fingers that will not straighten
- Nodules or hard bumps in the palm
- Fingers that pop or click; may or may not be painful
- A large bump that is present on the back of the wrist; may be painful
- Stiffness in the hands upon awakening
- Pains in the elbow

These symptoms are not always related to carpal tunnel syndrome and if you have experienced any of these symptoms it is possible that you are not suffering from CTS but a different condition. If that is the case, you need to speak to your physician so that a thorough exam can be performed in order to make a proper diagnosis of the condition.

It is quite likely that once a diagnosis has been made that your physician will be able to recommend a treatment program that will help to relieve the symptoms that are associated with the condition from which you suffer.

It is important to speak to your physician as soon

as possible, as putting off doing so will likely only lead to increased nerve damage, which could become permanent and irreversible, if left too long. The best course of action is always to address the situation as quickly as possible.

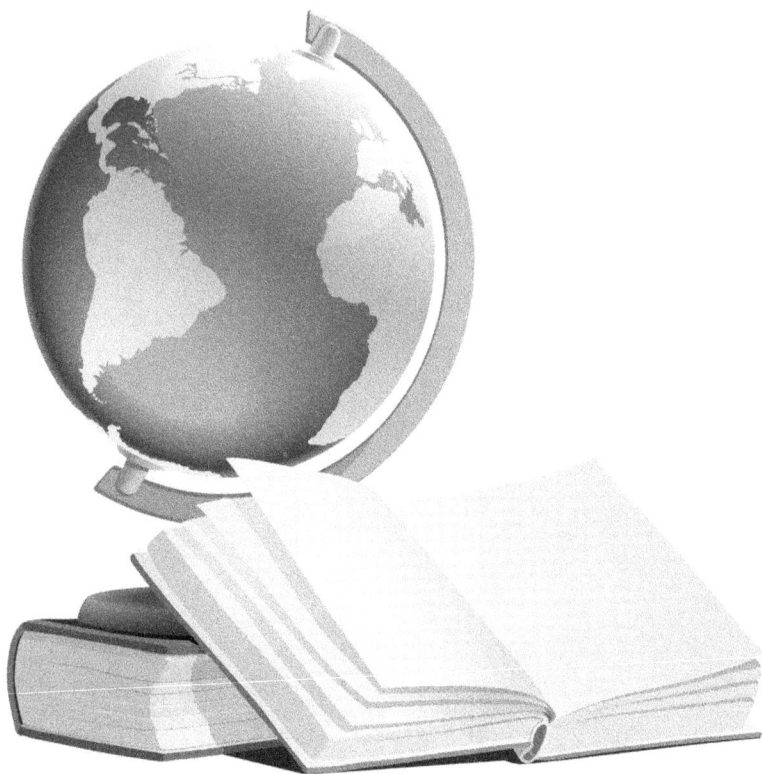

Glossary

The following definitions are meant to assist you in better understanding carpal tunnel syndrome.

Carpal tunnel
A small passage that is located below the wrist at the heel of the hand. The major nerve of the hand passes through this tunnel and is known as the median nerve. The tendons that bend the fingers also pass through here.

Cold laser therapy
A non-invasive procedure that utilizes low-energy or cold laser light to penetrate the skin and soft tissue

Dexterity
Refers to the skill and ease in use of the hands

Endoscopic surgery
A type of procedure in which fiber-optic tools are passed through a small incision in order to divide the transverse carpal ligament. This procedure is also known as keyhole surgery

Ergonomics
Refers to the science of matching a job and related equipment to individual human physical and psychological characteristics

Fibromyalgia
A chronic condition which can involve severe fatigue and involves the muscles and

connective tissue in which certain trigger points on the body become very painful.

Ligament
A band of fibrous tissue connecting bones, cartilage, and other structures

Median nerve
Conducts impulses from the brain, down the arm and to the fingers

Musculoskeletal
Referring to the muscles, joints and bones

Neurologist
A specialist in disorders of the central nervous system

Noninvasive
Refers to any procedure or treatment that does not invade the body through the use of insertion or incision

NSAID
Non-steroidal anti-inflammatory drug

Occupational medicine
The practice involving with injury and illness in the workplace

Orthopedist
A specialist in structural disorders of the skeleton, joints, fascia, muscles and other connective or supportive tissue such as

tendons, cartilage and ligaments.

Phalen test
Diagnostic test in which the wrist is bent forward for several seconds in order to see if CTS symptoms result.

Physiatrist
A specialist in physical medicine

Raynaud's disease
Vascular condition in which the fingers become pale and cold when blood vessels are constricted when exposed to cold

Repetitive strain injury (RSI)
An injury that is related to the upper extremities and results from prolonged overuse, force, pressure, awkward or constrained posture

Rheumatoid arthritis
Refers to a form of arthritis that affects the whole body.

Rheumatologist
A specialist in rheumatic diseases

Splint
A device that is used to immobilize a joint

Tendon
Fibrous tissue connecting muscles to bones and other parts

Tinel test

A diagnostic test in which the wrist is bent or pressed over the median nerve in order to determine if the tingling characteristics of CTS appear

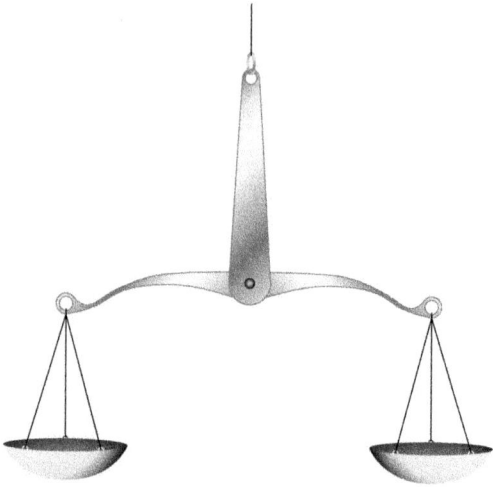

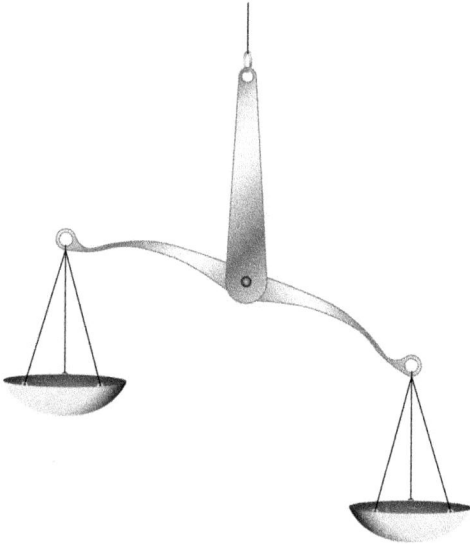

Conclusion

Carpal tunnel syndrome is a very serious condition which can result in painful symptoms and may restrict your daily activities as well as your ability to work, depending upon your specific line of work. There are many options for treatment that are available, including surgery and physical therapy. Not everyone responds to treatment in the same way. This is why it is imperative that you seek treatment as soon as possible in order to give yourself the greatest chance for recovery possible.

Other books by Psylon Press:

100% Blonde Jokes
R. Cristi
ISBN 978-0-9866004-1-8

Choosing a Dog Breed Guide
Eric Nolah
ISBN 978-0-9866004-5-6

Best Pictures Of Paris
Christian Radulescu
ISBN 978-0-9866004-8-7

Best Gift Ideas For Women
Taylor Timms
ISBN 978-0-9866004-4-9

Top Bikini Pictures
Taylor Timms
ISBN 978-0-9866426-3-0

Cross Tattoos
Johnny Karp
ISBN 978-0-9866426-4-7

Beautiful Breasts Pictures
Taylor Timms
ISBN 978-1-926917-01-6

For more books please visit:
www.psylonpress.com

www.ingramcontent.com/pod-product-compliance
Lightning Source LLC
Chambersburg PA
CBHW070933280326
41934CB00009B/1863